Part of You, Not All of You

Praise for *Part of You, Not All of You*

"Chronic illness changes all of your relationships, but the relationship impacted most of all is the one with yourself. This journal, compassionately guided by someone who intimately knows the ins and outs of forever sickness, gives chronically ill and disabled people the opportunity to write about their fears, hopes, grief, and joy. Most importantly, it offers the user a judgment-free space to explore what it means to live in an unpredictable and misunderstood body."

Tessa Miller, author of *What Doesn't Kill You: A Life with Chronic Illness—Lessons from a Body in Revolt*

"Living with a chronic illness does not come with a guidebook, but now, thanks to Jenneh Rishe, there is one. The author, who has candidly shared her struggles and triumphs with her social media followers, has crafted the perfect balance of a how-to book tempered with inspirational messages to help the reader throughout their personal journey. As someone with endometriosis, I would recommend this book to anyone with chronic illness as well as their loved ones."

Diana Falzone, journalist and endometriosis advocate

"Jenneh's unique book, *Part of You, Not All of You*, guides the reader through self-exploration. Journaling prompts encourage the reader to search one's inner depths to 'unpack heavy things' they are holding onto, to find self-worth, and to never forget that 'you are more than your illness.'"

Iris Kerin Orbuch, MD, director of the Advanced Gynecologic Laparoscopy Center and author of *Beating Endo: How to Reclaim Your Life from Endometriosis*

"*Part of You, Not All of You* is the right book at the right time for anyone facing health-related quality of life issues. Not just another wellness guide, *Part of You, Not All of You* centers on primary functions designed to empower patients who have one or more chronic conditions. It assesses needs, manages emotions and expectations, sets goals, and centers focus in order to encourage emotional, physical, and spiritual healing. Both informational and inspirational, this unique and practical guide meets readers where they are to help them plan, prioritize, and affirm their healthcare journey at their own pace and in their own way. *Part of You, Not All of You* is an essential resource for anyone seeking the support, encouragement, and indispensable tools necessary to triumph over adversities and optimize care as they navigate the chronic illness continuum."

Heather C. Guidone, BCPA, surgical program director at The Center for Endometriosis Care

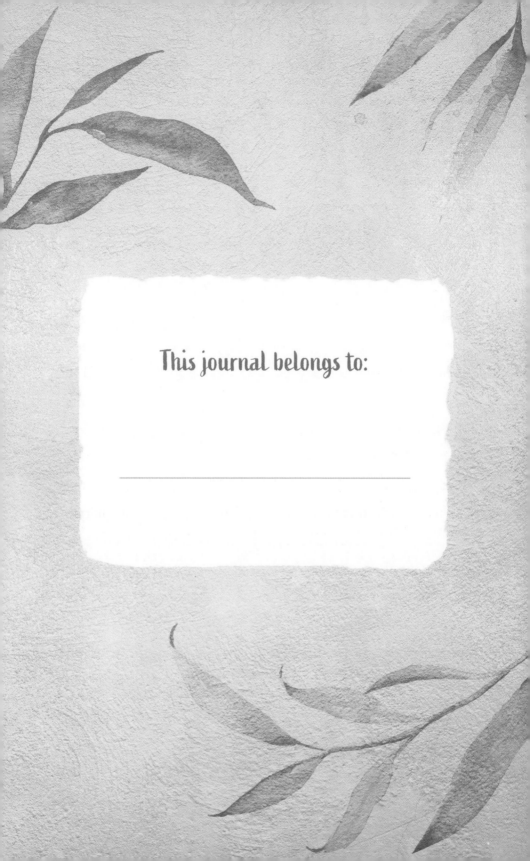

This journal belongs to:

_____

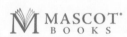

www.mascotbooks.com

Part of You, Not All of You: Shared Wisdom and Guided Journaling for Life with Chronic Illness

For more information, please contact:
Mascot Books
620 Herndon Parkway, Suite 320
Herndon, VA 20170
info@mascotbooks.com

Library of Congress Control Number: 2021916956

CPSIA Code: PRQ1121A
ISBN-13: 978-1-64543-784-0

Printed in India

Part of You, Not All of You

Shared Wisdom and Guided Journaling
for Life with Chronic Illness

JENNEH RISHE, BSN, RN

This book is dedicated to my
fellow chronic illness warriors.
You are stronger than you realize and
more resilient than you ever imagined.

Contents

Letter to the Reader

Dear whoever finds these pages,

I began my walk as a chronically ill woman at the ripe age of twenty-seven. Throughout my journey with multiple illnesses, journaling has been a staple of how I navigate the muddy waters of each new diagnosis. Writing things down on paper became instrumentally therapeutic in helping me process the many parts of my life that were constantly changing. I needed a way to chart a new path through relationships, friendships, identity, self-worth, and every other area of my life that was being affected by my illnesses. I needed a place to write down the things I couldn't always say out loud—the things that would sometimes keep me stuck in my own head.

Over the years, I've collected these reflections in different journals for different areas of my life: one for self-care, one for faith, and a blank one for all of my miscellaneous thoughts. Writing in these journals has given me the opportunity to dump all of my fears, desires, dreams, challenges, and triumphs onto their pages. And I've left each journaling session feeling a little lighter, like a weight has been lifted off me.

The words on these pages were written to help you navigate life with your illness and to encourage you to keep pushing forward when you need a little support. I hope this book will provide you a safe place to process it all, and will leave you feeling like you're walking through it with a friend. We may not know each other personally, but if this book is in your hands, there's a good chance we have many shared life experiences. The collective voices featured in this book belong to people who have shared these experiences too—people who have inspired me throughout my illness journey and have taken in stride, and with grace, the life they've been given.

Endometriosis, adenomyosis, infertility, heart disease, myocardial bridging, anomalous coronary artery, endothelial dysfunction, small intestinal bacterial overgrowth (SIBO), lupus, anxiety—this is the rainbow of afflictions I've been diagnosed with throughout the years, but they are not who I am. They

are part of me, but not the whole me. I am more than my illnesses, and I hope that by working through this book, you are
encouraged to accept the same truth: you are more than your
illness. So, so much more.

With love and light,

Jenneh

Benefits of Journaling

Journaling is often thought of as a form of self-expression, but focused journaling can also be a way to improve your quality of life. Some documented benefits of journaling include:

- Managing anxiety

- Reducing stress

- Helping prioritize problems, fears, and concerns

- Aiding in physical, emotional, and mental healing

- Boosting self-confidence

- Clarifying thoughts and feelings

- Helping define and achieve goals

Journaling has been an essential tool in understanding and managing my life as someone living with chronic illness. My hope is that *Part of You, Not All of You* will help you accomplish the same goal!

How to Use This Book

Part of You, Not All of You is divided into sections, guided by affirmations. Within each section you will find a collection of open-ended questions and list-type journal prompts, insightful words of inspiration from others who have embarked on their own chronic illness journeys, and words of encouragement and personal experiences of my own.

Throughout the book, you will notice opportunities for checking in along the way. These check-ins serve as a chance to center your focus on where you are in the present moment. You will be asked to assess your needs, set a goal (which can be as small as making your bed or as big as completing a project), name a highlight, and identify anything that is worrying or concerning you.

Lastly, you'll find some blank pages at the back of this book, where you can write about everything and anything you wish to put on paper. These blank pages can be used to dive deeper into a particular topic in the book, or to reflect on any miscellaneous thoughts you'd like to document. They're yours to use however you wish.

This book is meant to be worked through at your own pace, on your own schedule. I firmly believe that as people living with the daily demands of chronic illness, we don't need one more item on our list of things to complete—this book included! So there is no right or wrong way to work through it. One day, you may simply want an affirming word; another day you may want to dig deep. Either option is enough. The choice is completely yours.

However you decide to use it, I hope this book is something that you can keep coming back to—something to remind you of all you've conquered, who you are, and who you wish to become.

ONE

I Have Survived Every Challenge That Life Has Thrown at Me So Far

Write about your journey to being diagnosed.
What obstacles did you face?
Did you feel supported throughout the experience?
What was the most difficult part about it?

What is the most life-altering aspect
of living with your illness?

_____

_____

_____

_____

_____

_____

_____

List three negative things that have
happened as a result of your illness.

1.

2.

3.

Checking In

What are your mental and/or physical needs today?

_____

What is one goal you'd like to achieve today?

_____

What is one highlight of today or this week?

_____

What are your concerns, worries, or unknowns right now?

_____

Words of Inspiration

Erin White Robinson, YouTuber and digital producer

"During my struggle with fibroids and endometriosis, I learned that it's okay to give myself grace. For so long, I did not know that I was dealing with underlying health issues. I truly thought that every person dealt with a similar type of physical pain every day. I would beat myself up when I'd catch myself complaining about the cramps or the bloating or bleeding. I'd say to myself, *Everyone else is handling their own discomforts without moaning about it, Erin.* It wasn't until a doctor sat me down and explained things to me—that what I was going through was rooted in something clinical—that I began to give myself room to have those 'bad days.' On those days, instead of pushing myself harder to 'fake it,' I finally carved out time to allow my body to rest and recover.

"Our world has a tendency to praise and lift up people for portraying strength in the face of challenges. However, I learned that being strong isn't about looking strong to the world. Being strong is knowing when you're weak and loving yourself enough to get through to the other side.

"As for most people, my life has been a wild roller coaster of incredible peaks and extremely low valleys. When there are hard *I can't take this anymore* days, I actively force myself to close my eyes and walk back through my life's highlight reel in my head. I'm talking about the really big, big moments! I remember how miraculous it was that I was awarded scholarships for college, or how I was positioned at the right place at the right time when someone approached me to be on an amazing television show, or how I met my husband just weeks after a toxic breakup. I have to stop in the current moment and remember that just like before, beautiful and serendipitous days are bound to happen again, and this current moment will not last forever.

"Taking my mind to a place of gratitude always helps shift my perspective. Gratitude obviously doesn't make my pain go away, but it does remind me that whatever issue I'm walking through, it will pass, and a good day is bound to be around the corner."

TWO

I Give Myself Permission to Grieve the Life That I've Lost

What dreams have you had to put on
hold because of your illness?

_____

_____

_____

_____

_____

_____

_____

What do you wish people could
understand about your illness?

_____

_____

_____

_____

_____

_____

_____

_____

List three things you have lost and are
grieving as a result of your illness.

1.

2.

3.

Checking In

What are your mental and/or physical needs today?

_____

What is one goal you'd like to achieve today?

_____

What is one highlight of today or this week?

_____

What are your concerns, worries, or unknowns right now?

_____

Pivot When You Need To

Before I got sick, I had my whole life planned out. At the age of twenty-seven, I was a nurse manager at the Outpatient Cancer Center at UCLA Medical Center, and only three classes away from finishing my master's degree in nursing education at Drexel University with honors. Then, practically overnight, that entire plan dissolved right before my very eyes. I was forced to take a medical leave from my job for an entire year. It felt as though everything I had worked so hard for was being stolen from me, and I had no say in the matter. Plain and simple, I was lost.

Who do you become when you're stripped of everything you *think* you are?

My time of recovery also allowed for some time to soul search. My new body had its limitations that kept me from feeling confident enough to return to a rigorous work environment. But something else changed as well. After experiencing everything I experienced, I couldn't picture myself going back to pursuing the career path I was previously on.

My journey through chronic illness redefined my ideals and completely redirected my purpose. Chasing accolades and climbing a corporate ladder suddenly didn't seem so important. I was painfully confronted with my truth: it wasn't just about me anymore. I felt a new, overwhelming sense of purpose. So I made the decision to give myself grace and allow myself to play the hand that life had dealt me, which meant pivoting toward my dreams. And let's be clear: pivoting is not giving up. Pivoting from the path you felt you were destined for takes strength and immense bravery.

The life I'm living now isn't the life I dreamed of years ago, but it's not any less important or valuable. And maybe you're like me—trying to figure out what's next, searching for a new purpose or something else to identify with. Wherever you are in navigating *your* truth, know that there's someone out there who understands and is cheering you on so incredibly hard.

THREE

Putting the Pieces Back Together Takes Time

What are the most difficult challenges
you've faced because of your illness?

_____

_____

_____

_____

_____

_____

_____

_____

What gives you strength on tough days?

_____

_____

_____

_____

_____

_____

_____

_____

List three lessons that your illness has taught
you about life, yourself, or others.

1.

2.

3.

Checking In

What are your mental and/or physical needs today?

_____

What is one goal you'd like to achieve today?

_____

What is one highlight of today or this week?

_____

What are your concerns, worries, or unknowns right now?

_____

Words of Inspiration

Samantha Cohen, entrepreneur and advocate

"Living with a chronic illness, much of the time I feel like I'm on a rollercoaster. The constant ups and downs. The days that throw you for an absolute loop. The nights you get turned upside down. When, despite all your best efforts, you find yourself stuck riding over and over again. I wish I could end this analogy with a positive adage—'you will!'—or by me telling you, 'I've been there, and it gets better.' But the truth is I'm still there; I'm still riding.

"What I can say is a warrior's strength lies in their ability to stay there. Their resilience and unwavering resolve as they're being flipped on their heads. Faith, not in the medical community that has failed some of us, but in personal resolve, is what will keep you going. Some of us have been abandoned and hurt by those who we've trusted. It's a sad truth with chronic illness. Our strength must reside in ourselves and the communities we build. Our collective fortitude is of a different magnitude when those with chronic illness unite. We will get ourselves off of the rollercoaster one day, and we will bring each other along with us."

Words of Encouragement

"Today" is a word that I meditate on often. This short and simple mantra is a reminder that I have only enough energy and strength for the day that I am currently living in. While planning is a necessary part of life, when you're living with an illness, you don't always have control over what the day looks like—let alone what tomorrow has in store.

For some of us, even focusing on one day at a time can feel overwhelming. A good friend of mine shared a mantra with her husband during a particularly difficult season they were in: "minute by minute." Give yourself permission to take things day by day, minute by minute, or even second by second if that is what brings you comfort and peace.

FOUR

I Can Be Whole, Even If Parts of Me Are Still Healing

How can you show yourself grace on difficult days?

_____

_____

_____

_____

_____

_____

_____

The definition of "chronic illness" is lost on many people, even those full of good intentions who ask whether you're "feeling better yet." How can you best answer this question to give people a better understanding of what you're going through?

_____

_____

_____

_____

_____

_____

_____

List three boundaries you can put in place to protect your physical health as you continue the healing process.

1.

2.

3.

Checking In

What are your mental and/or physical needs today?

_____

What is one goal you'd like to achieve today?

_____

What is one highlight of today or this week?

_____

What are your concerns, worries, or unknowns right now?

_____

Heal at Your Own Pace, in Your Own Way, in Your Own Time

I know you've heard it time and time again: healing isn't linear. This idea applies not just to physical healing, but to mental and emotional healing as well. My own path to healing—whether it was navigating the medical trauma that came with having multiple illnesses, or processing the unexpected grief from learning I would never carry children of my own, or experiencing the long, painful, difficult recovery after open-heart surgery—has been up, down, left, right, and just plain crooked. Most of us would like to package our biggest hardships into a nice little box with a tag that says *HEALED* in big, bold letters, and never visit it again. I hate to be the bearer of bad news, but as I've learned through a lot of trial and error, that is not the way it works.

I liken my healing journey to climbing a mountain. Sometimes, the summit seems so close. At other times, I'm looking back at the base of the mountain and thinking, *It would probably be easier to just head back down.* Sometimes the setbacks are small, like a misstep when tripping over a rock. And at other times, the setbacks feel gigantic, like rolling headfirst down the mountain with nothing to break your fall.

I've found that, for me, healing has come in stages. Sometimes I revisit those stages even after I think I've already conquered them. Negative thoughts—like *We've been here before!* and *How are you not over this yet?*—start to creep in. Only when I realized that healing is not a checkbox life event, but a continuous journey, did my perspective begin to shift. Not every day was going to look exactly the same. One day I may be able to go for that hike, and the next day I might not. One day I may be totally okay attending a baby shower; the next day I might not want to go. One day I might be filled with anxiety at the thought of having to go to the doctor; the next day I might feel fine about it.

Naturally, the setbacks often come with major disappointment, but I try not to stay in that place for too long. I allow myself to feel frustrated, sad, angry—whatever I need to feel. But then I remind myself that setbacks and healing go hand in hand. I give myself the space to stumble and fall sometimes. I acknowledge that getting back up when I've been knocked down is the most courageous thing I can do. I speak positively to myself . . . to my body that has carried me through more than it ever should have been able to . . . to my mind that is still curious and open to change . . . and to my heart that is still soft, even though everything that life has thrown at it could have turned it into stone.

FIVE

I Am Worthy, Despite Any Physical or Mental Limitations I Might Have

What do you like most about yourself?

How can you show yourself kindness?

_____

_____

_____

_____

_____

_____

_____

_____

List three areas of your life, unrelated to
your illness, where you find self-worth.

1.

2.

3.

Checking In

What are your mental and/or physical needs today?

_____

What is one goal you'd like to achieve today?

_____

What is one highlight of today or this week?

_____

What are your concerns, worries, or unknowns right now?

_____

Words of Encouragement

Despite how you may feel sometimes, your illness does not make you any less worthy of love, acceptance, empathy, and understanding. You are worthy of being treated by others with patience and kindness. You deserve to enjoy two-way friendships, other fulfilling relationships, and virtually any good thing that life has to offer.

SIX

My Internal Healing Is Part of My Journey to Freedom

Imagine you had to write a letter of encouragement to yourself. What would it say?

_____

_____

_____

_____

_____

_____

_____

_____

What makes you feel most loved or cared for?

_____

_____

_____

_____

_____

_____

_____

List three boundaries you can put in place to protect your mental health as you continue the healing process.

1.

2.

3.

Checking In

What are your mental and/or physical needs today?

_____

What is one goal you'd like to achieve today?

_____

What is one highlight of today or this week?

_____

What are your concerns, worries, or unknowns right now?

_____

Words of Inspiration

Lacy Nicole, stylist, philanthropist, and health advocate

"I think with illness comes a lot of self-reflection. You learn to give others more empathy, even when you haven't always received it. The blessing in illness comes when you harness your power and realize your strength. I've found that connecting with others who go through the same hardships as you is a bond beyond measure. On both the bad and good days, I am encouraged by my faith and knowing God has a plan. I believe He gives us hardships to equip us to potentially help others."

SEVEN

Saying "Yes" to Myself Sometimes Means Saying "No" to Others

In what ways have you put other
people's needs before your own?

_____

_____

_____

_____

_____

_____

_____

How can you effectively communicate
your needs to those around you?

_____

_____

_____

_____

_____

_____

_____

List three things you'd like to learn to say "no" to.

1.

2.

3.

Checking In

What are your mental and/or physical needs today?

_____

What is one goal you'd like to achieve today?

_____

What is one highlight of today or this week?

_____

What are your concerns, worries, or unknowns right now?

_____

Choose Yourself

It was a Tuesday evening, and I was contemplating whether my symptoms were "bad enough" to go to the emergency room. When it became clear that the pain wasn't something I wanted to ride out at home, I threw in the towel and drove myself to the local hospital at 5:30 p.m. After hours of tests and observation, I was released at three in the morning. And what did I do next? I set my alarm for 5:30 a.m. so I could go to work because I had a presentation to give. I was so afraid of letting my team down that I completely put myself on the back burner.

This is an extreme example of not saying "yes" to myself, but I have many smaller examples that added up over time: agreeing to plans and events that I knew I had no strength for, working too much and too late, taking on other people's problems when I could hardly handle my own. I always felt guilty when I even considered saying "no" to anything. I worried about what others would think if I chose to take care of myself first—so I never did. As you can imagine, living this way led to a deep resentment within me. I felt like I was never able to catch a break. I was always looking for a moment to come up for air, but those moments never came. How could they? I didn't give them the space to surface.

Putting yourself first is considered selfish, but that is often a misconstrued belief. Maybe it's selfish when it comes from a place of self-importance and arrogance, but what if it comes from a place of self-preservation, self-improvement, self-care, or self-love? Showing up for yourself is never selfish. Taking care of yourself is never selfish.

There is a saying I've always loved, and it's among the truest sayings I know: "You can't pour from an empty cup." When you stop to think about it, prioritizing your needs is arguably one of the most *unselfish* things you can do. It is completely necessary in order to be the best version of you—not only for yourself, but for the people and things you care about most.

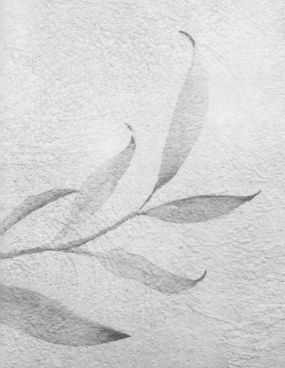

EIGHT

Needing Extra Support Does Not Make Me a Burden

How have you changed your behavior based on other people's feelings about your illness?

_____

_____

_____

_____

_____

_____

_____

When you are in physical or emotional pain, how does it affect your interactions with others?

What do you wish people could understand
about the invisible aspects of your illness?

_____

_____

_____

_____

_____

_____

_____

_____

List three people who have supported you throughout your illness, and describe how they supported you.

1.

2.

3.

Checking In

What are your mental and/or physical needs today?

_____

What is one goal you'd like to achieve today?

_____

What is one highlight of today or this week?

_____

What are your concerns, worries, or unknowns right now?

_____

Words of Encouragement

The people who are meant to be in your life will meet you exactly where you are. They won't force you to be something that you are not. Instead, they will encourage you to grow in unimaginable ways. They will walk with you until you get to the other side of your heartache. They will celebrate your wins and sit with you through your losses. They will listen and respond from a place of love and empathy, even if they don't fully understand. They will show you the same love that you show them. They will add to your healing instead of distract from it. They will help you see how much value you bring to the world. They will let you know that you are always enough, and never "too much."

NINE

I Will Look Back on Difficult Times to Remember How Far I've Come

What gives you hope?

It can be difficult to see how far we've come—
until we look back at where we've been. What is
something (big or small) that you are able to do now
that you couldn't do before, or that you thought
you'd never be able to do again? How would
you describe the feeling of accomplishment?

_____

_____

_____

_____

_____

_____

_____

List three things that encourage you to keep moving forward after a difficult day.

1.

2.

3.

Checking In

What are your mental and/or physical needs today?

_____

What is one goal you'd like to achieve today?

_____

What is one highlight of today or this week?

_____

What are your concerns, worries, or unknowns right now?

_____

Words of Inspiration

Alaia Baldwin Aronow, model and endometriosis advocate

"Through my illness, I have learned how strong I am—stronger than I ever could have imagined. I've gained perspective on what is truly important in life and how to focus on the positive. On my worst days, I try to remind myself that it's only temporary, and there will be more good, pain-free moments. On the good days, I try to be present and treasure each and every second. I have a much deeper appreciation for life's moments."

TEN

I Will Run My Own Race and Not Compare My Own Healing to Others'

What is most important to you in your life?

_____

_____

_____

_____

_____

_____

_____

_____

It can be hard to know when you're pushing yourself—both mind and body—to your limits. What are some ways to create a balance between overdoing it and pushing yourself beyond your comfort zone?

_____

_____

_____

_____

_____

_____

_____

List three short-term goals you have set for yourself.

1.

2.

3.

Checking In

What are your mental and/or physical needs today?

_____

What is one goal you'd like to achieve today?

_____

What is one highlight of today or this week?

_____

What are your concerns, worries, or unknowns right now?

_____

Words of Encouragement

If you're anything like me, you may find yourself comparing your own life journey to other people's journeys. Comparison has a tendency to rob us of joy and diminish our very real progress. Among the many reasons to stop comparing yourself to others, here are just a few:

- Your story is uniquely yours and no one else's.

- Your path does not have to look like the next person's.

- Just because something worked for someone else doesn't mean it has to work for you.

- Contentment is easier to come by when it's based on what *you* have instead of what others have.

- The value you bring to this world is immeasurable.

ELEVEN

I Will Allow Myself to Dream New Dreams, as Success Might Look a Little Different in This Season

What do you feel is your life's purpose?

_____

_____

_____

_____

_____

_____

_____

_____

What is something you've always wanted
to do that you've been afraid to pursue?
What holds you back from pursuing it?

_____

_____

_____

_____

_____

_____

_____

_____

List three long-term goals you have set for yourself.

1.

2.

3.

Checking In

What are your mental and/or physical needs today?

_____

What is one goal you'd like to achieve today?

_____

What is one highlight of today or this week?

_____

What are your concerns, worries, or unknowns right now?

_____

Words of Inspiration

Shannon Cohn, filmmaker and activist

"Yes, at times I've felt overwhelmed by my symptoms, but I've managed to not let them take over my life. I've made a point to keep up with professional and personal goals—some take days, weeks, or even months to accomplish. It's slower going, but the goals are still there. They keep me moving forward in endeavors unrelated to my illness and provide the necessary balance so I can be more than my illness."

TWELVE

It's Okay to Take a Break—Resting Is Not a Sign of Giving Up

Between appointments, medications, treatments, and self-care routines, living with an illness can feel like a part-time job. What practices can you put in place to help prevent burnout?

_____

_____

_____

_____

_____

_____

_____

List three healthy coping mechanisms that you practice.

1.

2.

3.

Checking In

What are your mental and/or physical needs today?

_____

What is one goal you'd like to achieve today?

_____

What is one highlight of today or this week?

_____

What are your concerns, worries, or unknowns right now?

_____

Speak Truth to Your Lies

There are times when I need tangible reminders of truth to drown out the lies swirling around in my head. It's not humanly possible to think positively all the time, and sometimes I unknowingly convince myself of lies that then take root in my mind. I have to remind myself: yes, I have limitations that are frustrating and sometimes overwhelming. But are those limitations the truest things about my life as a whole? Absolutely not. Is it true that I may need more rest than the average person? Yes. Does that fact make me lazy or inadequate? Not in the least.

Sometimes the lies masquerading as truths are so loud, there's only one way to remind myself that they are indeed untrue: by posting Post-its throughout my house. So if you ever come visit me, rest assured you're likely to find an encouraging note taped to my bathroom mirror, such as: "You've come out on the other side more than once." They offer a concrete visual to remind me of who I am, what I deserve, and where to fix my thoughts.

In a culture where overworking, overplanning, exhaustion, and burnout have become the norm, it's hard not to see rest as some form of weakness. At times, I've feared that resting was synonymous with me waving my white flag and saying, "I'm too weak to keep doing this." I let myself believe that lie for far too long. It has taken daily reminders to see that it couldn't be further from the truth. Honoring the truth about my need for rest means I can't say "yes" to everyone. When I stop trying to be everywhere and do everything, I can start thriving in the way my body and mind truly deserve.

THIRTEEN

I Am Not Defined by My Failures or Setbacks

Acceptance has been one of the most difficult parts about my chronic illness journey. Before my open-heart surgery, I would force myself to exercise, no matter how uncomfortable it was. I needed to prove to myself that I could still identify as a runner, even though at that time, I was not. I was stuck in a place where my mind refused to accept the fact that my body could no longer serve me the way it used to.

What about your illness journey are you
having a difficult time accepting?

_____

_____

_____

_____

_____

_____

What experiences have you let define you?

_____

_____

_____

_____

_____

_____

_____

List three things that make you doubt your capabilities.

1.

2.

3.

Checking In

What are your mental and/or physical needs today?

_____

What is one goal you'd like to achieve today?

_____

What is one highlight of today or this week?

_____

What are your concerns, worries, or unknowns right now?

_____

Words of Encouragement

You are not defined by the worst things you've done, the mistakes you've made, the biggest success you've achieved, the tasks you complete, or how busy your calendar is. Instead, see yourself in the way you show kindness, the way you positively affirm yourself, and the way you seek joy. Focus on the way you triumph over hardships time and time again, and the way you keep fighting for yourself. Let those attributes shine as brightly as they deserve to, because they are the most beautiful things about you.

FOURTEEN

I Am Strong Even If I Question, Fear, or Doubt

What is your greatest fear? How can
you work toward facing this fear?

_____

_____

_____

_____

_____

_____

_____

_____

Will I ever get better? is a question that has often kept me up late at night. How does the uncertainty of your illness make you feel?

_____

_____

_____

_____

_____

_____

_____

_____

List three things related to your
illness that cause you to fear.

1.

2.

3.

Checking In

What are your mental and/or physical needs today?

_____

What is one goal you'd like to achieve today?

_____

What is one highlight of today or this week?

_____

What are your concerns, worries, or unknowns right now?

_____

Words of Inspiration

Jillian Schurr, attorney

"Although my illness has made me stronger, I've learned that the tough exterior—which I was known for prior to being sick—was truly just an exterior. I learned to feel things I often used to shut off. By opening the door to those emotions, I was able to fuel my passion to survive and advocate. I remind myself that even with my illness, being debilitated and confined to bed, I still have so much to contribute to the world. My illness will never stop me."

Define Your Own Version of Strength

"You are so strong." If I had a dollar for every time I've heard this over the past several years, I could probably retire on a private tropical island. Do not get me wrong—being told how strong I am is a huge compliment. Yet at times, it has made me feel like the biggest fraud. Are "strong" people in therapy to work through their problems? Do "strong" people burst into tears and sob while sitting at traffic lights, hoping the stranger in the next car doesn't notice? Do "strong" people question whether or not getting out of bed today is actually worth it?

The narrative around strength can be a rigid, unrealistic one. It tells you to hide your pain and put on a smile that you don't really mean. It tells you not to admit your struggles and says that falling apart is not an option. It forces you to say "I'm fine" when nothing could be further from the truth.

I have worn my "You are so strong" badge with honor. But attempting to live up to being "strong" has sometimes kept me from growing, feeling, experiencing, and most importantly, healing. When I faced some very big moments in my life, being "strong"—at least in the way the world views strength—was not an option. One example is when I had to sign a consent form for my open-heart surgery and acknowledge that one of the possible risks was death. Was I supposed to remain "strong" in that moment? Or was I allowed to sit with the very real possibility that I might never see my mother and my husband again?

Admitting that I was terrified may not have appeared strong, but I know now that strength does not always show itself in the traditional sense of the word. Asking for help when I need it—that's strength. Continuing to advocate for myself when test results came back inconclusive was also strength. And strength also is admitting that I do not have all the answers. Letting others in and sharing the most intimate details about my life is definitely not for the weak. Realizing when I've mentally and physically pushed myself to my limits is strength personified. Accepting my flaws is strength too.

I will gladly accept the "You are so strong" compliment any day. But I have chosen to redefine what strength looks like for me. I wear this new badge with even more honor than I wore the old one.

FIFTEEN

I Will Remember That Progress Is Still Progress, Even If It's Small

What do you consider to be a "productive" day?

_____

_____

_____

_____

_____

_____

_____

In what ways have you pivoted in your life,
given the challenges you've faced?

_____

_____

_____

_____

_____

_____

_____

List three people to whom you look for inspiration.

1.

2.

3.

Checking In

What are your mental and/or physical needs today?

_____

What is one goal you'd like to achieve today?

_____

What is one highlight of today or this week?

_____

What are your concerns, worries, or unknowns right now?

_____

Words of Inspiration

Dr. Akilah Cadet, MPH, founder and CEO of Change Cadet

"Living with a heart condition—with the daily pain, endless appointments, and medications—I've learned that I am amazing. I am able to live my life to the fullest, even with a broken heart. I actually don't think much about 'good' days. I am very 'in the moment' at all times. Early on, when I was, like, 'I'm having a good day,' within an hour that would change. I would get a horrible heart spasm. So now, I just do what brings me joy. If that means working out, great. If it's binging on a show, great. If it's crying, great. I focus on joy.

"As a result of my diagnosis, I am able to be my true, authentic self. I have to be more transparent, as I have an invisible illness—and with that, I've become able to be transparent about everything. The best compliment I receive is when someone says I'm my true, authentic self."

SIXTEEN

I Will Create Room for the Things That Help Me Heal, Grow, and Learn

How have you remained "you" despite your illness?

_____

_____

_____

_____

_____

_____

_____

_____

What does the practice of self-care look like for you?

_____

_____

_____

_____

_____

_____

_____

_____

List three things you would like to forgive yourself for.

1.

2.

3.

Checking In

What are your mental and/or physical needs today?

_____

What is one goal you'd like to achieve today?

_____

What is one highlight of today or this week?

_____

What are your concerns, worries, or unknowns right now?

_____

Words of Encouragement

For some time, I believed that self-care required me to actively partake in some sort of relaxing ritual, such as applying a face mask, taking a bath, or reading a magazine. I was often left feeling like I didn't have the time, energy, or space to practice self-care as I understood it. But what if I told you that self-care can be accomplished without *doing* so much?

At its core, self-care is simply about taking care of yourself in ways that allow you to be the best version of yourself. Self-care doesn't have to look only like rest and relaxation. Sometimes, self-care shows up in the form of simply allowing yourself to feel everything that you need to feel.

SEVENTEEN

I Am Deserving of Relationships That Allow Me to Be My Authentic Self

How has your illness changed your
relationships in a negative way?

_____

_____

_____

_____

_____

_____

_____

How has your illness changed your
relationships in a positive way?

_____

_____

_____

_____

_____

_____

_____

Describe a time when someone showed you
empathy. How did it make you feel?

List three qualities that you look
for in a good friendship.

1.

2.

3.

Checking In

What are your mental and/or physical needs today?

_____

What is one goal you'd like to achieve today?

_____

What is one highlight of today or this week?

_____

What are your concerns, worries, or unknowns right now?

_____

Foster the Healthy Relationships You Deserve

Let's talk about navigating relationships with chronic illness. For starters, we should break it down into three main categories: family, friends, and romantic relationships. These relationships are all uniquely different—they have different dynamics and different expectations.

When it comes to family, your expectation may be an assumed unconditional alliance. That may not always be the case. You might find that a complete stranger is more supportive than a family member has been.

When it comes to close friendships, your expectation may be that friends will meet you where you are with understanding. Yet you may discover that some of your closest friends have been the least understanding.

When it comes to romantic relationships, your expectation may be love. Sometimes, though, the person who loves us simply does not know how to love *all* of us.

I had a difficult time in all three of these areas.

I count my lucky stars that I have an incredibly supportive family. Their support for me has always been unwavering. Where I found myself in trouble was my inability to be completely honest with them, for fear of letting them down or putting too heavy a burden on them.

I pride myself in always having it all together. I was always the person to whom others would go for help or advice, not the one seeking help. I didn't want my mother, who lives three thousand miles away, to stress over me. I convinced myself that it was best for my family not to know just how sick I actually was. Until things got "really bad," why make anyone worry unnecessarily?

Well, things got really bad, really quickly, to the point where I wasn't even capable of working anymore. Only then did I share my entire truth with my family: my illness had consumed me, and I needed their help. They stepped up in every way that I needed them to, by offering me support physically, emotionally, and even financially at times. In the entire year that I was on medical leave from work, my brother—who is unarguably my best friend on this planet—did not go a single day without calling, texting, or FaceTiming me. After my first surgery, my sister left her family in Chicago to be my nurse in Los Angeles for an entire week. My mother, whom I like to describe as an angel on earth, spent months at a time with my husband and me in our one-bedroom apartment, offering to do anything and everything we needed to survive. Looking back, I'm sure my family would have wanted to be there all along, pitching in. I just had to give them the chance.

Friendships were a whole other story for me. The fact of the matter is, many young adults have not yet lived through a life-altering experience. We are vibrant and believe we are untouchable. Our body not working the way it's supposed to—that just isn't on our radar. So, among my friends, there was a learning curve in figuring out how to be a good friend to me in this moment. There was a learning curve for me, too, in figuring out what I expected from a friendship in this new season of my life.

Becoming sick forced me to take inventory of whom I surrounded myself with. Who made me feel most comfortable when I shared with them? Who made me feel uncomfortable? Who made it easy for me to be real, honest, and authentic?

Who meant it when they said they would always be there for me? Who made me feel guilty when my symptoms forced me to cancel plans? There were difficult conversations and even more difficult decisions. And yes, there were some friendship casualties—not everyone made the cut.

Ending a friendship is never easy, even if there is good reason. But from the other side, I can honestly say now—for the first time in my life—that the people who are around me today are people I can count on in the most difficult times. I know they will be there lifting me up, encouraging me, and supporting me. Our relationships are not one-sided. These are what I consider true, lifelong friendships.

But I wish someone had written a manual on how to tell your new boyfriend that you have a chronic illness, because I definitely could have used one. This, by far, was the most complicated relationship for me to figure out. I happened to meet a really great guy just two months before my diagnosis of endometriosis. Talk about bad timing! I didn't tell him much about my disease. The only reason I brought it up at all was because I felt so horrible during a flare-up that my doctor ordered me to take a week off from work, and I had to give my boyfriend an explanation.

I made it seem like it wasn't a big deal. Honestly, what would I even say? Leading with the truth—"I know we've only been dating for a few seconds, but I have this debilitating disease that keeps me up every night in pain, may mean I can't have children, and has no cure"—didn't seem like the best option. Let's be clear: we all have our baggage. But when is it too soon to unload your baggage onto someone else?

I knew that it was my body, and my choice whether to share or not, but I also felt dishonest about leaving out the major details of a very big aspect of my life. I had to give him the choice of loving me through something he had absolutely no experience in.

We had one good month together of me being "well." After that, every day was consumed with doctors, surgeries, and everything else that comes along with chronic illness—and he chose to continue walking with me through it. We fast-forwarded through the getting-to-know-you dating phase and jumped headfirst into survival mode.

I remember one particular day, two months into our relationship, I was on the floor sobbing. One of my new medications was making me emotionally unstable. My now-husband said to me, "I don't know who you actually are, because you are a different person every day, but I have a feeling it's worth sticking around to find out." I am so glad that he did. He showed me that the right person will meet you exactly where you are, help you sort through all of your mess, and give you the room to become who you're meant to be.

I am not the same person I was five years ago when this

journey first began. I've lost parts of me that needed to go, and I've uncovered pieces that I never knew existed. I guess that's what suffering does to you: picks you apart and makes you decide what version of yourself you're going to be left with. The dynamics of all of my relationships changed as I emerged, a brand-new me—someone who was forever changed by my lived experiences, and whose relationships reflected this in all the best ways.

EIGHTEEN

I Am Capable of Showing Myself Patience, Love, Honesty, and Respect

What are some self-limiting beliefs that you
have about yourself? How do these beliefs keep
you from achieving what you're capable of?

List three areas in your life where you
could show yourself more patience.

1.

2.

3.

Checking In

What are your mental and/or physical needs today?

_____

What is one goal you'd like to achieve today?

_____

What is one highlight of today or this week?

_____

What are your concerns, worries, or unknowns right now?

_____

Words of Inspiration

Joseph Rishe, software developer and filmmaker

"As strange as it sounds, dealing with depression gave me some advantages. Maybe most important, it gave me the courage to make difficult changes in my life. I moved across the country to escape winter and left everything I knew behind. I changed a job that was adding to my depression. I even changed careers entirely, to something I was more passionate about. Without the deep reflection that depressive episodes brought on, I don't think I would've had the courage or clarity to do these things. Yes, my illness is a burden, but positive things have come out of it."

NINETEEN

I Will Put Down Yesterday's Burdens and Focus Only on My Needs for Today

What future burdens are you carrying with you today?

_____

_____

_____

_____

_____

_____

_____

What helps you remain present in
the events of the current day?

_____

_____

_____

_____

_____

_____

_____

List three things that you would like to let go of.

1.

2.

3.

Checking In

What are your mental and/or physical needs today?

_____

What is one goal you'd like to achieve today?

_____

What is one highlight of today or this week?

_____

What are your concerns, worries, or unknowns right now?

_____

Words of Encouragement

Trying to remain positive and look for silver linings in the face of uncertainty is helpful in getting through trying times. But this can be really hard when the what-ifs blur out any visions of hope. With this in mind, I have come to three conclusions:

1. It is completely okay to try to remain positive yet still have moments of frustration.

2. It is completely okay to grieve while you're working toward acceptance.

3. It is completely okay to cling to hope yet still feel hopeless at times.

These positive and uncertain feelings are not mutually exclusive. Life is not a series of "either/or" situations. Life is a collection of "and also" realities.

TWENTY

I Can Set Myself Free from Other People's Expectations of Me

We've been conditioned to believe that most people would like to keep conversations light and airy, so you may wonder: when someone asks how you're doing, do they really want to know? Because of this, many of us carry our burdens on our own. Even when we do find others with whom we are comfortable sharing, it can be difficult to find that fine line between what feels like being honest and what feels like oversharing.

How comfortable are you discussing your illness with others? What barriers keep you from sharing personal details?

Do you think people see you for who
you truly are? Why or why not?

_____

_____

_____

_____

_____

_____

_____

_____

List three people you know you can share
with, without fear of judgment.

1.

2.

3.

Checking In

What are your mental and/or physical needs today?

_____

What is one goal you'd like to achieve today?

_____

What is one highlight of today or this week?

_____

What are your concerns, worries, or unknowns right now?

_____

Allow Others to See You for Who You Really Are

The unpredictability of living with a chronic illness was one of the most challenging things for me to work through. Never knowing how I would feel at any given moment played an unexpected role in my life in many ways. Ultimately, it led to paralyzing fear and deep insecurity. I was afraid to meet new people, because I feared they wouldn't understand my life. I was afraid to pursue dreams, because I feared having to quit if my symptoms became unmanageable. I was afraid of making plans, because I hated having to cancel at the last minute. I was afraid I would never find a life partner, because I feared no one would accept me with all of my baggage.

To me, these fears were all very rational, and I was justified in feeling every single one. I was entitled to sit and make sense of them for however long I needed to. But even if they were rational, the truth is, these fears led to me feeling isolated and alone. I had unknowingly put my entire life in a box, one that allowed my illness to determine every aspect of what I did and how I felt about myself. I felt the need to hide so many aspects of myself that I was practically living a double life. There was "sick" me, and then there was "pretending-not-to-be-sick" me. I preemptively decided that no one would understand me and my world, so I never bothered to explain.

The problem with this way of thinking is clear to me now. On one hand, I craved compassion and empathy from others. On the other hand, I never gave anyone the opportunity to be empathetic and compassionate toward me. Instead, I would make palatable excuses that didn't even scratch the surface of what I was actually going through. Why? To prevent myself from experiencing any letdown or disappointment. To avoid disappointing other people or making anyone feel uncomfortable. And this meant my needs were not being met, my relationships were not genuine, and I had no sense of who I truly was.

Over time, I realized that the root of my fears could be

boiled down to this: the unpredictability in my life made me highly insecure, which made me fearful of any situation that would "expose" the real and complicated aspects of my life. I learned that authenticity is hard to come by when, knowingly or unknowingly, you are keeping parts of yourself hidden away. I discovered that I was no longer willing to allow my insecurities about my illness to keep me from living a truly authentic life.

TWENTY - ONE

I Choose to Focus on What I Can Do Versus What I Cannot Do

Think about a time when you felt joy. What
were you doing? Whom were you with?

_____

_____

_____

_____

_____

_____

_____

How can you make more room for the things
in your life that bring you happiness?

_____

_____

_____

_____

_____

_____

_____

_____

List three things that instantly help shift your mood.

1.

2.

3.

Checking In

What are your mental and/or physical needs today?

_____

What is one goal you'd like to achieve today?

_____

What is one highlight of today or this week?

_____

What are your concerns, worries, or unknowns right now?

_____

Words of Inspiration

Meghan Maloof Berdellans, real estate/relocation specialist,
marketing consultant, and The Endo Co board member

"When you're chronically ill, it can be easy to lose yourself. Prayer, meditation, and daily positive affirmations have been critical in keeping myself grounded and allowing me to always remain my true self. Every morning, I write down three things I am grateful for in order to start the day with a positive mindset. Health is always in my top three. Health is wealth, and the time best spent is with people you love and care for. Never take any moment for granted."

TWENTY - TWO

I Will Make a Conscious Effort to Let Gratitude Lead Me Through My Day

What is your definition of happiness?

_____

_____

_____

_____

_____

_____

_____

What areas of your life bring you happiness?

List three things that you are grateful for.

1.

2.

3.

Checking In

What are your mental and/or physical needs today?

_____

What is one goal you'd like to achieve today?

_____

What is one highlight of today or this week?

_____

What are your concerns, worries, or unknowns right now?

_____

Words of Encouragement

Positivity is a great thing. Toxic positivity, on the other hand, is not. Toxic positivity tells you to keep a mentality of "it could be worse" and "look at the bright side" and "good vibes only." When you're going through trials, being told to "stay positive" can feel incredibly unhelpful. Being positive 100 percent of every day, in every circumstance, isn't realistic or healthy; it diminishes very real feelings that you are entitled to feel, and it can lead to downplaying issues that instead deserve time to process and work through. Sometimes seeing the light at the end of the tunnel feels impossible, and you shouldn't feel forced into always seeing life through rose-colored glasses.

What I am a fan of, though, is practicing gratitude. I've gotten into the practice of naming one thing a day that I am grateful for in my life. Even on my worst days, I can come up with one thing. Sometimes it's as simple as being grateful for the sun shining!

To practice gratitude, I don't have to pretend that life is perfect. Gratitude allows me to hold the negative and positive side by side. Practicing gratitude doesn't ask me to completely block out any negative emotions. Instead, it gives me the freedom to shift my thoughts, even if it's only for a moment, to things that bring me peace and comfort.

TWENTY - THREE

I Will Focus Less on My Physical Imperfections and More on the Beautiful Ways I've Continued to Bloom Through Brokenness

What do you believe are your best qualities?

_____

_____

_____

_____

_____

_____

_____

At what time or moment in your life have you felt most comfortable in your own skin?

_____

_____

_____

_____

_____

_____

_____

_____

List three positive personality traits that
others have used to describe you.

1.

2.

3.

Checking In

What are your mental and/or physical needs today?

_____

What is one goal you'd like to achieve today?

_____

What is one highlight of today or this week?

_____

What are your concerns, worries, or unknowns right now?

_____

Show Love for Yourself—Every Single Part of You

Life with chronic illness brought myriad physical changes that appeared out of the blue and were out of my control. The medication side effects, such as inflammation and weight gain, made it difficult for me to even recognize myself in the mirror some days. The actual symptoms of my diseases made me look pregnant in a matter of seconds if I ate something my body didn't agree with. And then there were the physical scars. I could feel strangers staring at the remnants of multiple abdominal surgeries when I'd wear a bathing suit. I saw the look of pity when the eight-inch scar down the center of my chest caught someone off guard.

The psychological changes, too, took me by surprise: the self-doubt from being gaslit by medical professionals . . . the trauma of worst-case scenarios playing out repeatedly . . . the sadness and anxiety that came as a package deal with uncertainty and the unknown. Looking at me, you wouldn't know that I struggled with any of these insecurities. On the outside, I carried a self-assuredness that did not match my interior. Meanwhile, my internal dialogue constantly criticized me; I was too complicated, too damaged, too scarred to be considered worthy. So I overcompensated by trying to portray a picture of perfection, which was harmful to both my mental and physical health.

How could I ever expect anyone to see me as worthy if I didn't see myself that way? My self-limiting beliefs were holding me back. Constantly pretending to be someone else was not sustainable, and I knew deep down inside that I needed to do something about it.

My thoughts were powerful, and they shaped how I viewed and cared for every part of me—especially the parts I didn't love. I was able to admit that I *liked* myself, but I didn't truly *love* myself. I was not showing myself the same understanding, acceptance, and compassion that I showed others. And as a result, my self-esteem and self-worth were severely suffering.

This is where making a mindful, intentional effort to show self-love came in. It began with something that may sound a lot easier to practice than it actually is: positive self-talk. What did this mean, exactly? It meant that the way I spoke to myself was just as important as the way I allowed others to speak to me. It meant that I wouldn't speak words to myself that I would never say to a friend. It meant the harsh self-criticisms had to go.

Practicing self-love has been an ever-evolving exercise for me. It is one that I need to practice daily. I have to forgive myself for my mistakes. I must agree to show myself patience. I surrender to my flaws. And I vow to accept my physical and emotional scars. Instead of viewing them as negative and shameful, I see them as a beautiful roadmap of everything that I have lived through.

TWENTY - FOUR

I Will Let Myself Fully Enjoy Moments of Hope, Happiness, and Good Health

If you could recreate one moment
in time, what would it be?

_____

_____

_____

_____

_____

_____

_____

_____

What do you keep in mind on your "good days"?

_____

_____

_____

_____

_____

_____

_____

List three things that greatly influence
the happiness in your life.

1.

2.

3.

Checking In

What are your mental and/or physical needs today?

_____

What is one goal you'd like to achieve today?

_____

What is one highlight of today or this week?

_____

What are your concerns, worries, or unknowns right now?

_____

Words of Inspiration

Leslie Mosier, creator of Doug The Pug

"If it weren't for endometriosis, I would have never known my inner strength of being vulnerable. This illness has caused me to open up in ways I never thought possible—not only to people on the internet, but to my friends and family and, most [importantly], my husband. It has taught me how to communicate and how to ask for help when I need it most. It has opened me up spiritually and truly catapulted me into my spiritual journey and desire to know myself more. I lean on my husband and our animals a lot. My pug always knows when I am in pain. I practice gratitude and do a lot of self-love affirmations. I am grateful for my body, even when it is hurting!"

TWENTY - FIVE

I Am Greater Than the Sum of My Accomplishments

What do you feel is unique about yourself?

What is the one thing you are most
passionate about? Why?

_____

_____

_____

_____

_____

_____

_____

_____

List three things that make you proud of yourself.

1.

2.

3.

Checking In

What are your mental and/or physical needs today?

_____

What is one goal you'd like to achieve today?

_____

What is one highlight of today or this week?

_____

What are your concerns, worries, or unknowns right now?

_____

Words of Inspiration

Jahmby Koikai, creative artist and broadcaster

"Living with a chronic illness has taught me that there's a warrior in each of us. The best advice I can give is to find your support system. These are the people that you trust and can count on while navigating the challenges that present themselves. It may be family, friends, or other supportive communities. My family has always been by my side and [has] been a constant source of emotional and physical strength. Most importantly, I encourage you to keep faith alive that you will get through the storm."

TWENTY - SIX

I Can Take Comfort in Learning to Release the Things That Are Out of My Control

How does not having control over
your health make you feel?

_____

_____

_____

_____

_____

_____

_____

What do you feel in control of in your own life?

_____

_____

_____

_____

_____

_____

_____

_____

List three things you can do to simplify your life.

1.

2.

3.

Checking In

What are your mental and/or physical needs today?

_____

What is one goal you'd like to achieve today?

_____

What is one highlight of today or this week?

_____

What are your concerns, worries, or unknowns right now?

_____

Words of Encouragement

What purpose does this serve? is a good question to keep in the forefront of your mind to help you focus on the things that push you forward. You're struggling with so many things that feel completely out of your control. On top of that, expectations placed on you by others (sometimes unknowingly) can feel like the weight of the world on your shoulders. Set your boundaries and limits. Choose what's most important. Your mind and body will thank you.

TWENTY - SEVEN

I Can Find Joy in Each Day, Even If It's Just for a Moment

What "little things" do you find joy in?

What would a peaceful day look like for you?

_____

_____

_____

_____

_____

_____

_____

_____

List three barriers that keep you from experiencing joy.

1.

2.

3.

Checking In

What are your mental and/or physical needs today?

_____

What is one goal you'd like to achieve today?

_____

What is one highlight of today or this week?

_____

What are your concerns, worries, or unknowns right now?

_____

Enjoy the Ordinary

I'm a list maker. I'm a task checker-offer. I'm a planner. For most of my life, I found idle time incredibly uncomfortable. If I wasn't planning something or doing something, I honestly didn't know what to do with myself. I was always on the go. I was constantly double-booked. A full calendar was brag-worthy to me. My brain was always ten steps ahead of my body. I was always rushing from one thing to make it to the next thing. I was almost never fully present.

I would now describe myself as a recovering over-doer. Reflecting on the past, most of my days feel like a blur. I never sat still long enough to soak in what moments of happiness actually felt like. I admit, part of my busyness was a defense mechanism. Being busy kept me from having to acknowledge all the ways my life was falling apart.

A lot changed when my entire world was forced to stop. I could no longer partake in the things I once thought of as mundane—things that I once took completely for granted. Only in looking back do I realize that I wasn't actually *living* my life. I was merely passing through it.

Today, my appreciation for the seemingly ordinary moments in life could not be greater. Moments like going to a new coffee shop . . . taking a walk down my favorite street and noticing how beautiful the flowers are . . . having a lazy Saturday with my husband, when our only agenda is to binge-watch our favorite show. Suddenly, every moment of joy feels so much sweeter, no matter how temporary it is. Suddenly, every conversation deserves my full attention. Suddenly, hearing my favorite song on the radio fills me with more warmth than ever before.

My calendar has a lot fewer plans in it these days. My to-do list is shorter than it used to be. But I can assure you, my life is fuller than I ever could have imagined.

TWENTY - EIGHT

A Promising Future Is Still Within My Reach

If you could make one major contribution
to the world, what would it be?

_____

_____

_____

_____

_____

_____

_____

What does the word "contentment" mean to you?
What areas of your life make you feel content?

_____

_____

_____

_____

_____

_____

_____

_____

How can you practice living a life of contentment?

_____

_____

_____

_____

_____

_____

_____

List three personal values that you
try to live your life by.

1.

2.

3.

Checking In

What are your mental and/or physical needs today?

_____

What is one goal you'd like to achieve today?

_____

What is one highlight of today or this week?

_____

What are your concerns, worries, or unknowns right now?

_____

Words of Inspiration

Julian Gavino, social activist

"One of the biggest things chronic illness has taught me is patience. I used to be a person who angered rather quickly. When you're disabled, you have to wait for everything—a wheelchair takes months, doctor's appointments take hours, a diagnosis can take years . . . the list goes on. I really value the peace I've found in patience. It hasn't been an easy road, but learning patience has allowed me to apply it to other areas of my life. I notice I'm a lot more patient with other people and more empathetic than I used to be. I don't cry over spilled milk. I just let go and trust the process. Because whether I want a process or not, it's there.

"If anything, I'm more me than I've ever been. I feel blessed that through my transition and illness, I've been able to see multiple perspectives that no one else has seen. I wouldn't be me without my experiences, and those experiences led me to my purpose. It can be really hard—none of it is easy—but after you accept it, things can get easier in a sense. You find your people. You find ways to cope. There's nothing I can do about it, so why not make the best of it? I truly believe my soul's mission in life is to fight for diversity, inclusion, and disability rights."

TWENTY – NINE

I Am Enough, Just as I Am

What negative phrases do you use
when speaking about yourself?

_____

_____

_____

_____

_____

_____

_____

_____

What positive phrases can you replace
the negative phrases with?

_____

_____

_____

_____

_____

_____

_____

_____

List three people who make you
feel accepted, just as you are.

1.

2.

3.

Checking In

What are your mental and/or physical needs today?

_____

What is one goal you'd like to achieve today?

_____

What is one highlight of today or this week?

_____

What are your concerns, worries, or unknowns right now?

_____

Words of Encouragement

Being a work in progress is worth celebrating. It means there is still abundant room to become the person you feel called to be. You will continue to grow. You will continue to learn. You will continue to uncover parts of yourself that you love and parts of yourself that are coming undone. You will continue to shed layers of pain, regret, and grief. Through it all, be encouraged and be generous with yourself. Settle into being an unfinished project. Embrace being a perfectly imperfect human being. And in the meantime, allow yourself to accept that you are enough, just as you are.

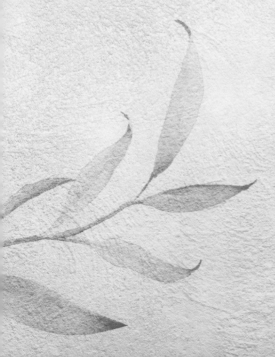

THIRTY

I Am More Than My Illness

How has your illness shaped the
way you view the world?

_____

_____

_____

_____

_____

_____

_____

_____

What has happened to us does not have to define *who we are.* A chronically ill thirty-four-year-old who has had a hysterectomy, a thoracic surgery, three abdominal surgeries, and open-heart surgery in just four years is what *happened* to me, but it's not *who I am.* Has it influenced the person I've become? Yes—but it's not my identity.

It takes a conscious effort to not let your circumstances rob you of who you are or what you aspire to be. Whether it's sickness, a personal failure, a broken relationship, a traumatic experience, or something else—you are so much more than these things.

How would you describe yourself to
someone you have never met?

List three things unrelated to your illness
that have helped shape your identity.

1.

2.

3.

Checking In

What are your mental and/or physical needs today?

_____

What is one goal you'd like to achieve today?

_____

What is one highlight of today or this week?

_____

What are your concerns, worries, or unknowns right now?

_____

Words of Inspiration

Khalida Outlaw, registered nurse and actress

"I've remained 'me' by constantly reminding myself that I *have* endometriosis, but I *am not* endometriosis. This chronic disease does not define my entire being. Despite the inconveniences, extreme pain, hospitalization, surgeries, and multitude of scars, I am still a beautiful, intelligent, talented, funny, compassionate, sexy-a** Harlem girl with a multitude of blessings."

Believe Your Illness Is Not All That You Are

There was a time when my illnesses were very much my entire life. I was completely wrapped up in them. They consumed most of my waking thoughts—and rightfully so. My illnesses *are* a huge part of my life. They affect things like the amount of planning and coordinating that goes into seemingly simple tasks like choosing what to eat for breakfast, whether or not I should drive today, or how to come by sleep more easily tonight. The reality of being sick means not having the luxury of putting my illnesses in the back of my closet, to be brought out at a more convenient time.

I also acknowledge that at one time my illnesses occupied an unhealthy portion of my identity. I found myself describing who I was as *someone with [insert list of diagnoses]*—endometriosis, SIBO, heart disease—more than anything else. And though these truly were parts of my identity, I was leaving out huge parts of who I was. Spending so much time in the wilderness of chronic illness, I had forgotten who I actually was before my diagnoses.

Processing my loss of self was similar to experiencing grief: I went through denial, anger, bargaining, depression, and finally, acceptance. Acceptance, for me, meant releasing the idea that I would ever be exactly who I was before my illnesses. This might sound like a sad and somber thing. But over time, it wasn't. Acceptance meant recognizing that my illnesses will always be a *part* of me, but they are not *all* of me.

I didn't magically arrive at this place of acceptance. No. Not even close. This process slowly took shape as I chipped away gradually at years of hurt, disappointment, and what I thought of as betrayal by my own body.

Once I finally found myself at this place of acceptance, I realized that even though I couldn't control the circumstances of my life, I could control my outlook. I could control my attitude. I could control how I chose to see my worth and identity. And I chose not to define myself only by my diagnoses, because I'm much, much more than that. I am a nurse

... a wife ... a daughter ... an author ... a sister ... an entrepreneur ... an aunt ... a good friend ... a believer ... and the list goes on.

Now, for the first time in my life, I can say I *truly* know who I am. I'm aware of the parts of me that still need to heal, and I give space to the parts of me that still need room to grow. I don't push myself beyond my limits to make others happy. I celebrate every win, big or small. I forgive myself for the days I'm unrealistically hard on myself. I surrender to the reality that there will be hard days ahead, and I do my best not to let my setbacks take away from the very real progress I've made. I still have days when I feel the immense weight of living with chronic illness—I would be lying if I said I did not. The difference is, I'm finally in a place where I refuse to let those days make me question my worth or doubt my purpose. I won't let the difficult moments define my existence.

I don't think I will ever get to a place where I can say I'm thankful for my illnesses, but I will say I'm thankful for who I've become because of them. In a way, they've shaped my favorite things about myself and my life: my empathy for others ... my ability to look for the good in impossibly hard situations ... the deep relationships I've formed ... my relentless determination ... my hope to live a full life despite difficult circumstances ... my gift for connecting with people ... my journey of self-exploration ... and my desire to see people for exactly who they are.

Could I have arrived at a place of being my true self without going through such heartache and pain to get here? Possibly. But I cannot deny that everything I have lived through has played a significant role in who I am today—someone I am proud to have gotten to know. Someone who is more than her illnesses.

I am so honored to have been on this journey with you so far. I hope that working through this book encouraged you to unpack some heavy things that you were holding onto, or discover something new about yourself. If nothing else, I hope this book helped you realize that you are not alone—that there is someone out there who knows where you are. I hope you feel seen, loved, accepted, and heard. I hope you realize how much you have to offer to this world, despite the tough circumstances you've encountered.

And most importantly, I hope you never forget that you, too, are more than your illness.

Use these pages to write about anything
else your heart is carrying.

_____

_____

_____

_____

_____

_____

_____

_____

Resources

I know firsthand that living with a chronic illness can sometimes feel really isolating. I want to remind you that you don't have to do it alone. There are incredible individuals, organizations, and communities creating spaces and resources for you to feel empowered, supported, and seen. Here are a few of my trusted favorites!

- Chronicon: www.thechroniconcommunity.com

- Mighty Well: www.mighty-well.com

- Chronically Capable: www.wearecapable.org

- Path to Empowered Acceptance with Natalie Kelley: www.plentyandwell.com

- Coaching and learning community of support with Rosemarie Philip, PCC: www.rosemariephilip.com

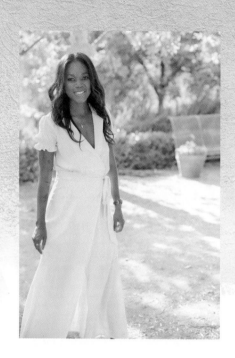

About the Author

Jenneh Rishe has been a registered nurse for more than a decade, working in several different specialty areas such as surgical trauma, oncology, and internal medicine. She is the founder of The Endometriosis Coalition, a nonprofit organization with a mission of spreading awareness, promoting reliable education, and increasing research funding for endometriosis.

With her love for healthcare, education, and teaching, Jenneh felt inspired to use her expertise and personal life experiences to help others gain a better understanding of their health while also offering hope and encouragement along the way. Through the years, Jenneh has become an advocate for the endometriosis and chronic illness communities. Her advocacy work and personal journey have been featured in various media outlets such as *Women's Health* magazine, *Vice News*, *Cosmopolitan*, *Darling* magazine, *Healthline*, and *The Today Show*.

Jenneh is originally from New Jersey but has lived in Los Angeles for the past ten years. In her free time, she loves running, writing, soaking up the California sun, and spending time with her incredibly supportive husband, family, and friends.

Connect with Jenneh

Personal website: www.jennehrishe.com
Instagram: @lifeabove_illness
Twitter: @JayAreRishe
LinkedIn: www.linkedin.com/in/jennehrishe
The Endometriosis Coalition website: www.theendo.co